BIODYNAMICS OF OSTEOPATHY

Pediatrics Two

Second Edition

James Jealous D.O.

For more information about Dr. Jealous please visit:
https://BiodynamicsOfOsteopathy.com

BIODYNAMICS OF OSTEOPATHY   Pediatrics Two

Hardback ISBN: 979-8-2955-3936-7

Second Edition 2025

James Jealous D.O. (1943–2021) practiced as an osteopathic physician, teacher and writer for many years. His life's work was to found and develop the specific methodology of Biodynamics of Osteopathy, following the lineage of Dr. A.T. Still and Dr. W.G. Sutherland.

This is one of a series of Biodynamics of Osteopathy books. They grew organically from sets of handouts written by Dr. Jealous and given to students during courses taught by him and his teachers. After many years he collected the handouts together and created individual course manuals, which he added to and rewrote many times. After several more years they evolved further into books.

TABLE OF CONTENTS

OSTEOPATHY IS SERVICE viii

IMAGES OF THE HEALTH FROM STILL AND SUTHERLAND 1

THE NORMAL CHILD 6

PERCEPTUAL STUDIES: THE FLOW OF THE ATTENTION 10

THE STUDY OF THE ACTIVITY OF ATTENTION 12

AT THE CENTER OF OUR BEING 13

COMMUNICATION 14

PEDIATRICS TWO: SKILLS REVIEW 16

NEUTRALITY 18

PEDIATRICS PHASE TWO: OVERVIEW 21

DIRECT AND INDIRECT METHODS IN THE TREATMENT OF CHILDREN 24

ZONE B AND THE THREE LEVELS OF STILLNESS 26

THE PELVIC BOWL AND THE PERINATAL PERIOD 29

THE PRENATAL PELVIS 32

THE PASSAGEWAY 33

FETAL MALPOSITION, TURNING BABIES 34

THE PERINATAL PELVIS 37

PRACTICAL APPLICATIONS 39

THE PERINATAL PELVIS, PART TWO 41

THE PELVIS 44

MEDITATION 45

THE DESERT NEUTRAL 47

REVIEW OF TREATMENT OF CHILDREN 49

NEUTRAL 50

COMMUNICATION 52

REMOLDING THE CHILD 54
DOORWAY BETWEEN ZONE B AND THE OCEAN 55
CHILDREN'S SENSORIUM 56
MEDITATION 58
A MEDITATION FOR PRENATAL WOMEN 60
QUOTES FROM SEVEN- TO NINE-YEAR-OLD CHILDREN 61
KEY POINTS 65
BREATHING IN CHILDREN AND ADULTS 67
CHILDREN AND PRIMARY RESPIRATORY DYNAMICS 70
THE WHOLE PATIENT 72
BREATHING AND CHILDREN 73
THORACIC RESPIRATION AND PRIMARY RESPIRATION IN CHILDREN 75
THE FIRST BREATH 76
THE WHOLENESS 79
NEITHER/NOR 83
BASICS IN THE TREATMENT OF CHILDREN 84
THE PERCEPTUAL JOURNEY TO THE MEETING PLACE 88
CHILDREN AS ONE 89
ALL THE CHILDREN WHO WILL NEVER BE TREATED 90
A CHILD'S SENSE OF WHOLENESS, THE FAMILY CIRCLE 91
WHOLENESS 92
MAINTAINING A TREATMENT 93
THE FAMILY CIRCLE ... PERSONAL MEDITATION 94
POTENCY AND FIRE 95
BIODYNAMICS OF OSTEOPATHY BOOK SERIES 97
ABOUT THE AUTHOR 103

OSTEOPATHY IS SERVICE

We use our hands ...

To treat the Whole patient

To listen to the indwelling movements of Life

To treat all levels of illness

To assist in building the patient's functional reserve

To support homeostasis and trophicity by balancing the activity of the autonomic nervous system

To explore "laws not framed by human hands" (Dr. Still and Dr. Sutherland)

To cooperate and communicate with the Laws of Nature (Dr. Wales)

"To find the Health" (Dr. Still)

To get to the treatment plan

To get to the diagnosis

To help establish a point of Rest or Neutral around which the Whole can come to balance

To find Cause

We believe ...

We have an innate capacity to heal

The patient functions as a whole

The autonomic nervous system plays a major role in disease and healing

Structure and function are one form of activity

The Divine is indwelling

Life moves beyond death

There is a Constant Movement toward Normal

We are here to Serve Humanity

Normal is ...

"A sense of peace and harmony" (Dr. Sutherland)

Ease of motion, without tension

A capacity for Neutral

A sense of Wholeness to Life

The capacity for adaptation, change without compensation.

"Skill is proportionate to one's understanding of normal" (Dr. Still)

"Eternity is a child playing…"

–Heraclitus

IMAGES OF THE HEALTH FROM STILL AND SUTHERLAND

"Children Are Transparent to the Health" These Words Are Paramount to the Treatment of Children in the Biodynamic Method.

Certainly Dr. Still posed a very profound truth when he said, "Find the Health; anyone can find disease." ... What does this mean? ... What is it like to experience the Health in oneself and others ... Has anyone described it?

Drs. Still and Sutherland both describe an experience of the Health.

At eighty-six years old, Dr. Still said, "I love my patients. I see God in their faces and their form."

These words are not timid. Dr. Still was straightforward. He was not looking at lesions. How did he come to this "ability"? I do not know.

I can report on how this has happened for myself and thousands of other osteopaths—practitioners who do see the Health, the Divine, and movement of life in their patients.

My introduction to this approach was from Dr. Rollin Becker personally, and in his 1965 Sutherland memorial lecture about the spiritual fulcrum, he states, "The Deity centers us." This refers to the Divine centering us ... it is not us who center ourselves. This awareness is common in contemplative practices that appreciate our inner poverty. "It is by the grace of God that we can perceive the invisible work of the Spirit." There is a distinct awareness when this happens to us. We are transformed in seconds from our own content to being an effect of another deeply loving presence. Our effort must have ceased in order for us to see the moment of impregnation and a total change in being.

Still was clear that human intelligence has severe limits without the intercession of a higher mind.

To witness the health in another person, one's senses must be transmuted by the Health itself, touching one's being when one is Neutral. This was made clear to me by Rollin Becker, when he looked at me one day and said, "Do not begin your treatment until the will of the patient surrenders to the will of Primary Respiration." He was very direct and concrete as he said this. I was shocked. He had taken the end point of treatment as I understood it and made it the beginning. After many years his guidance became clear and profound.

The treatment begins when there is a sustained Neutral in the Whole. Children have this most of the time. Even sick children are transparent to the Health. This transparency is a special kind of Neutral that is persistent in children, in spite of their disease. Children do not lose their capacity to love, even when they are critically ill. Adults, as you know, change their moods with their sense of wellness. You will find that even very ill children will center you. They transmit the flow of the Divine.

When we are in a Neutral that is saturated with Third Level Stillness, we become receptive in a unique manner. We are Neutral, waiting serenely for the Tide to enter the moment and unveil to the senses the invisible world of the Health. This is the "deity centering us," creating a new level of awareness. In working with children, because they are deeply suffused by the Divine and the incarnate Health, their mere presence is enough to "center" us and bring our senses to "seeing" the Health ... if ... we are Neutral and at the "Meeting Place," i.e., the Third Level of Stillness.

This requires an inner awareness of the many ways we can fool ourselves.

Our senses operate from the self-centered mind of our self-image. What does this mean? The synapses in our brain develop around familial and cultural interchanges. As children and young adults, we have many projections placed on us. From these trillions of synapses, we form a synthetic center ... one we created from the world around us, not the one in us from the beginning of life.

Many of us are working to "find our health and discover ourselves" as we were originally made. That is to say, "To see God's face and form in ourselves and others," as Dr. Still stated.

Our senses, and ourselves, are attached to the ego, and so we see others as projections of our own classifications, not as transparent beings, reflecting the Divine image of the Health. We are all doing this. This understanding helps us to understand neutrality and to make a choice to allow "Deity to center us" ...

Children will do this for us ... if we meet them at the Meeting Place. The transparency of a child to the Health allows the Health to come out into the world, and those who are able will respond by being "centered by the child" ... then we are able to see the Health in others.

One sees the world as transparent and Whole. The sense we have of a child is that they are "empty" and transparent to the movement of creation. We see a transcendent love entering through them, "creating/healing" the cellular unfoldment of the child.

This appreciation of a simple and clear awareness of creation is part of the legacy we receive from Drs. Still and Sutherland. Let's review their teachings.

Dr. Still refers to "mind, motion, matter."

Dr. Still said that these laws are not "framed by human hands."

The mind he speaks of is the Supreme Intelligence of the Divine Mystery. This Mystery animates as the Breath of Life (i.e., motion) which incarnates as the material world (matter). Thus we have Spirit, moving into creation, and unfolding the blueprint of life. We can see this if we are "centered by the Tide." When centered we can see mind, motion, and creation as a singularity of the movement of life as a Whole.

The sensation of eternity entering time is beauty.

Sutherland and others follow the lead of Still.

In the first edition of Magoun's *Osteopathy in the Cranial Field,* Sutherland reports both his view and Still's view of the Health, "a transparent Wholeness without systems or parts." Remember, this is not philosophy but the report of direct perceptual activity.

"...Motion must be guided by a Supreme Being, down to the individual cell, otherwise there would be chaos and death." (A. T. Still)

Sutherland then quotes Still further:

"Dr. Still understood the cerebral spinal fluid as the highest known element in the human body; he envisions this fluid as an intermediary in the movement of divine intelligence ... a channeling of creation into embryological segments and irrigating them with life ... giving form and function, order and intelligence to our existence. All life is manifest in his motion" (see page 15, paragraphs 1 and 2).

This is what we see when we awaken to the Health...

In *Contributions of Thought,* Sutherland again addresses a simple picture of Wholeness (see April 12, 1948).

Here Sutherland describes feeling the cerebrospinal fluid and the Breath of Life (the movement of Supreme Intelligence) ... feeling the spark of life that ignites the potency. An unerring, overshadowing, and superseding function that he called Primary Respiration.

He sees a dynamic interchange (Becker) between creation and the created ... These impressions came to Sutherland only after he stopped using force!

Later in life, Dr. Sutherland asked his wife to paint a picture of Primary Respiration as he experienced it. Again, another image appears that mimics those we have just discussed. The painting is called "A House Under the Sea."

This painting was lost in political bickering, but the story has been told to me by three of my mentors, Ruby Day, Anne Wales, and John Harakal. Recently, I was told by a historian that the house in the painting was A. T. Still's cabin ... that would suggest a very deep love and remembrance of his teacher.

The "house under the sea" is biodynamic in the sense that this image is similar to Blechschmidt's insistence that we are formed from a mysterious force coming through us from the "outside." The similarity with Still, Sutherland, and the foundation of osteopathy in embryology is what prompted me to choose the name "Biodynamics of Osteopathy." The commonality of images provoked by all these observant men is heartwarming to anyone who has felt these things and feels "a little crazy" when told that there is only structure in osteopathic diagnosis and treatment.

The image of a house, transparent to the "ocean of the Breath of Life," brings again the sensory experience of transparency. Of "something" passing through us unimpeded, that heals/creates as it passes without diminishing itself. This Supreme Intelligence is the master mechanic, the physician within the Health, the higher self, and the Divine image in all of life.

Children are the archetype of normality, radiant with these truths.

Our elders saw these truths ... we can approach their teaching only when we are Neutral and free to be centered by Deity ... this is why we call it "the Meeting Place."

THE NORMAL CHILD

The following observations, in part or in whole, can be made of a normal child. Diagnostics can be accomplished by following these guidelines. By noticing the qualities noted here, one will often find a disease process before it completely unfolds. This is the hallmark of osteopathy and preventive medicine. Traditional diagnostics on children are limited and do not "see" problems until it is "too late."

A child that recovers from an illness is not "cured" until these qualities reappear.

Being at Third Level Stillness creates the receptivity to perceive these things.

Transparency. The Imago Dei is visible. Children radiate the Health as if they were translucent. They feel like "a House Under the Sea" suffused by the Tide.

Self-Remembering in Adults. When a child comes into our presence, it creates a memory of our own health. We have a recollection of a deep presence behind life. This feeling connects us with a different kind of memory. If this does not happen, find out why ... is the child restrained somehow ... look carefully.

Children Are Healers. If a child physically touches you or looks at you with a gaze of intent, you will feel a communion and healing. Often, the depth exceeds any that we witness in osteopathic treatment.

Zone B Is Translucent. Children have no Zone A. The presence of even a small area of A is an alarm, telling us to look deeper into the cause.

Innocence. A normal child makes no calculation of loss when following the movement of creation ... when the Spirit moves, so moves the child.

Free Will. Children have a unified experience of love ... a freedom to respond without reservation. If this is missing, we must find out why … it is very important to the child's growth and health.

An Awareness of Belonging to God. There is a good overview of this in *The Spiritual Life of Children* by Robert Coles. If you are not aware of this quality in children, then I recommend the book.

Children Feel the Movement of Creation. This language comes from Phase Eight. It means that a child feels the movement of eternity, somatically. As adults, we very rarely feel this. It is the "now" that mystics like Eckhart Tolle speak about. Creation did not end. It continues.

Children Are a Wholeness. This is a fact that diagnostics can overlook. The growth of a child is done as a whole, not in parts. There is only one fulcrum for the expression of involuntary motion (i.e., growth, primary and secondary respiration).

Children Are Wise. Again, if this is unfamiliar to you, read the book by Robert Coles.

If the above qualities fade or are missing, find the cause.

They Live in the Unfolding of the New. There are several points to observe here. First, a child is not aware of the next new quality to arise, and yet they step into it fearlessly. They adapt and begin to sense this new quality with joy. Adults are not even looking for change. Children live on the limit of their understanding and reach for more every day. Adults rarely exceed their limits. Children explore the unfoldment with passion. Children also look for the source of the "newness" … they will search and find the fulcrum. Once a normal child finds a garden hose and plays with it a short time … that child will find the faucet and make the cognizant connection to the source of the water. This is rapid in a normal child. The exploration is driven by the intelligence of the Whole, unfolding.

A Normal Child Has Unconditional Love.

One Breath. Normally, the Primary and Thoracic Respiration are one with the movement of the Whole.

A Divine Gaze. A normal child will look "far away" and stop, filling with Holiness. When they look at you, you may feel the same.

Becoming Connected to Third Level Stillness. When adults in the immediate environs are consciously aware of Third Level Stillness, a normal child will respond. A report I received on a case highlighted the importance of this. A severely ill child was not responding to treatment as we expected, from what the Tide was showing. The clinician made a house call ... taught the family about Third Level Stillness, and the response to treatment was greatly accelerated! This fact is food for children.

Rest. Children rest. This is a key quality. If it is missing, find the cause.

Suffering Is Suffused with Love. When children are sick, they do not separate from the Health. Very ill children are still porous to the Health.

They Are Charitable. Children often give away their "best" possessions.

They Are Direct. The end is the end.

A Normal Child Loves Animals.

They Have Faith. A normal child is comfortable with mystery.

They Have Imagination. A child should be imagining. Psychologists often think that imagination is a fantasy; it is not. Again, please read Dr. Coles's book. Imagination was recognized by Dr. Sutherland as an asset for adults in understanding Primary Respiration. The word "imagination" was originally identified as "the highest form of intellect." Today, it is a word misused and dead to its real meaning. The art of daydreaming is lost.

Joy

Playfulness

A Oneness with All Children

These are qualities to observe in the child to see if they are "normal," from a functional osteopathic model. If any of these are missing ... find out why ... look for the cause ... before they develop a serious liability.

"Our skill is proportionate to our understanding of normal." ... Dr. Still has directed us to be noble in our discovery of what is normal, what it is like to be normal ... and children can help us a great deal.

PERCEPTUAL STUDIES: THE FLOW OF THE ATTENTION

Motion is the essence of life. This is the First Principle of Osteopathy. Where there is motion there is a natural direction toward Normality, Neutrality, and Wholeness.

Normal is a state of "peace and harmony," not necessarily a state free of disease. Neutrality is a state of freedom where one is moved involuntarily by the Health. Wholeness is a state of being where all "healths" are experienced as a singularity.

The state of our attention conditions what we perceive. As clinicians, we become aware of the liabilities involved in perceptions that are static, and how disease and pain are outcomes of static perceptual flow. Attention that is normal flows; it has intrinsic motion that is an expression of the Health.

Education and insecurity train the attention to converge,[1] to go to a place and hold there, stopping the natural flow and creating stasis, which causes the perception to separate from the Health. The result is loneliness and grief, often unseen.

The attention is a substance, an energy that flows from the Source of Life, and as such is naturally at work following the intention of the Breath of Life,[2] of Love, the Potency of Life, moving into manifestation in Eternity.

---

[1] Convergent and divergent language from Ken Johnson's YouTube video. Drs. Sutherland and Still stressed divergent thinking as the means of exploration into "laws not framed by human hands."

[2] See chapter 1 of the first edition of *Osteopathy in the Cranial Field*, and April 12, 1948, in *Contributions of Thought*.

When the attention is free to move, one does not feel time, death, or separation from anything, even enemies.

As osteopaths, I would hope that we are naturally interested in the "involuntary motion" that is guided by an unerring potency, an unfailing source of order and Wholeness. This teaching was a legacy that Dr. Sutherland carried forward in time for us. As we explore it, we will find that we do not necessarily believe osteopathic principles. It is normal to think that words are just ideas ... until you meet someone who lives the words and demonstrates their reality by "uncanny"[3] clinical results. Then, I believe we are obligated to our patients to dig on and explore ideas as realities, and see what the results are in our own practice.

My mentors challenged every technique I employed by asking me to change to using principles in practice. The work I had to do was severe ... hard. There were three big obstacles. One was that my practice was very successful and my clinical outcomes very good (not whole, but good). Another was that I like being an authority both in lecturer and mentor. It was exciting to "know" and be successful. Third, I was afraid of what I did not know, and protected it with false certainty. I was afraid of not knowing what was happening in myself and others.

The trust of my mentors was what ultimately allowed me to try out their methods and survive the fear of loss that naturally came with deeper principles. My life shifted for the better and the clinical results were dramatically better, which I thought was impossible. So we learn.

---

[3] *Uncanny* is a word Dr. Sutherland uses a lot to describe the supernatural healing effects of the Potency of Primary Respiration. These effects are completely out of the realm of expectations based on good clinical reasoning.

THE STUDY OF THE ACTIVITY OF ATTENTION

"Our skill is proportional to our understanding of normal." Dr. Still

Dr. Still's words will challenge us to look not at our capacity to find sessions and diagnoses, but to understand normal. To understand means to experience and know normal by seeing its motion and cause. Our first goal in studying the activity of attention is to "dig on" by observing it in ourselves, and later in others as we try to help them.

We begin by watching our attention, something we are not used to doing. What is it doing? Where is the fulcrum? What is the cause?

Is it flowing from inside to outside, freely or fixed? Where does it originate? All this we do by sensing the attention as it works, or as it locks up and lesions (stops flowing).

Let it flow to the interior of yourself. What does it do? Where does it flow? Does it stop on a thought or a feeling? Does it flow into a place?

As the day passes, every once in a while, try to see what your attention is doing and record the event. Remember, we are trying to understand normal; in other words, what does the attention do when allowed to express its truth, its motion?

AT THE CENTER OF OUR BEING

In *Conjectures of a Guilty Bystander* (1966), Thomas Merton writes:

> At the center of our being is a point of nothingness which is untouched by sin and by illusion, a point of pure truth, a point or spark which belongs entirely to God, which is never at our disposal, from which God disposes of our lives, which is inaccessible to the fantasies of our own mind or the brutalities of our own will. This little point of nothingness and of absolute poverty is the pure glory of God in us. It is so to speak his name written in us, as our poverty, as our indigence, as our dependence, as our sonship. It is like a pure diamond, blazing with the invisible light of heaven. It is in everybody, and if we could see it we would see these billions of points of light coming together in the face and blaze of a sun that would make all the darkness and cruelty of life vanish completely . . . I have no program for this seeing. It is only given. But the gate of heaven is everywhere.

COMMUNICATION

The teaching of osteopathy has always included, at its core, the effort to engage the natural laws of healing. This of course did not mean "laws framed by human hands" as both Still and Sutherland emphasized. Dr. Wales, who led our study group for over 30 years, repeatedly said, "Our goal is to communicate and cooperate with indwelling laws of healing."

The Fluid Body is a living intelligence that expresses growth and healing through a dynamic state of neutrality. It has a mind that precedes and creates the central nervous system. This means it has an organized intelligence that creates form, function, and tempo. It is not just a biological fluid that is an effect ... it makes the effects.

Our efforts to communicate with the Fluid Body reveal that the actual pressure or fluid drive is less than one millimeter of mercury. This suggests a remarkable tensionless field that baffles scientific thinking. This low-pressure theory is the result of studying venous pressure in the cranium.

Studies are hard to find, but the intracranial venous pressure is very low (2 mm). When you see a cranial bone and look at the interior surface, you can see the imprint of the venous sinus. This means that the fluid field making the bone is in balance with the low venous pressure. The venous channels are often said to invade the bone. This is misleading. There is no invasion. The venous system and the bone are both made from the same forces, indicating that the pressure in the whole is at a balance point. The system is remarkably poised.

What this means is that if one wishes to listen to the Fluid Body in a child or an adult, then the hands must be in a fluid Neutral, thus becoming part of a continuum.

How much pressure does it take to compress a vein on your hand? Try it. It seems very little, yet the venous pressure in the hand is much, much higher than that in the cranium.

This is an interesting topic to explore.

PEDIATRICS TWO: SKILLS REVIEW

The Spiritual Life of Children

We are blind to the perceptual world of children, yet we can become receptive to them and learn a great deal about communication and change.

Adults are monosynaptic compared to children. As adults, we choose less freedom and creativity than children do. Children are rarely distracted. They concentrate with a freshness and lack of anxiety about outcomes, which touches the world softly.

The book *The Spiritual Life of Children* by Robert Coles is interesting in that it begins with an attempt to prove that children have vivid imaginations due to a lack of perceptual maturity. The author discovers that there is a truth they perceive; however, nothing is ever learned about what they do experience. The children spiritually direct the author. The book is helpful. We can see what modern medicine is thinking and, as osteopaths, how differently our science appreciates the vision of children.

Wholeness is something that is a fact. As adults, we may appreciate this, but we do not necessarily experience it as the status quo of our perception. A child senses this Wholeness as an elemental essence in everything. They are wonderfully uniting and strive to pull us away from the partitions we feel to be necessary.

This simple understanding of Wholeness that we appreciate is spiritual. It expresses higher virtues and feelings. In embryology, the idea of Wholeness is slowly coming into view. The study of Neutral is in fact a study of Wholeness at different levels, the ultimate being when a patient feels as transparent as a child. Dr. Still focused on Wholeness. We as osteopaths spend a lifetime unraveling our lesions to clear our inner air of clouds. Wholeness has no politics; it includes everyone and every form of posture.

The study of different levels of Stillness is a journey into healing our adult attitudes. The Meeting Place is a Third Level Stillness. It is not where we meet the child, but where they meet us. We are a guest. In this place, their beingness heals us and illuminates our hearts so we can see more deeply into Primary Respiration and its intentions. Being a guest is not easy for most of us; we want to participate. What we do not see is that wanting to participate in this place, we are docile or Neutral. Neutral is empty of purpose; even the desire to be attentive to the child should not come from us. Neutral is neutral, peaceful, and empty of the desire to interact.

If you are interested in being rearranged, then work at neutrality.

NEUTRALITY

I would like to say a little about neutrality in oneself and how important it is to "being," in relationship with the Health in ourselves, others, and especially children.

Neutral, as Sutherland talked about it, was an automotive metaphor. When a car is in neutral, it is not engaged in any direction ... forward or reverse ... it just sits idling, with the engine running. In the ancient teachings, the metaphor about neutrality builds around oneself as a passenger, not the driver.

The driver is the master ... the car is our soma ... the direction of the car is Divine intention ... the journey is a mystery ... rarely do we know exactly where the car is going ... so we remain neutral even when activity begins. The hand of God moves the levers and the gears of the "mechanism" ... giving a sense of ease to the passenger in the car, who is in reality a guest, well served by the master. We do not take the wheel!

A mystic once said we should be blank. No anticipation, no plan, no understanding of "whither we go." I like this, but there is fire in the room. One is not blank of senses, only of will.

Neutral is a special room inside the "house under the sea" ... the room has no sense of humanity in it, either yours or others'. What is in the Neutral is purity, transparency, and a sweet, soft, inaudible joy that never leaves the heart to enter the world.

Neutral is a place where one can be free. It is a place where insult and injury are so meaningless that in their presence the joy increases. How strange this seems to our logic. What hurts the ego when one is Neutral adds potency to the spirit. What could wound us heals us.

Neutral is a holistic awareness. It is not "mine." There is no sense of my Neutral.

No one can see you unless they are with the Whole, so the projections flow, but the energy never comes in the room ... one is safe from one's ego as well as that of others.

It seems that Sutherland's affinity with Neutral grew from Still and his colleagues ... I feel from reading Sutherland that he was clearly taken in the Direction of Ease by Still's guiding hand, but then felt the need to go more direct until he matured (see *Contributions of Thought* and study Sutherland's perceptual odyssey).

The history of the idea of Neutral is as old as the oldest recorded history of man's quest for Wholeness (the Vedas) and as old as oral history (the African bushmen). It is a state of pure nonviolence and charity.

The three forces of yogic background are emblematic of the three states of Divine expression and are studied in oneself as a tool for approaching a union with God ...

In the Bhagavad Gita there is a battle between the positive and negative forces, but the master takes the student into the space between the duality to begin his teaching ... this is neutral ground.

The images of the three forces—active, passive, and neutral—are not to be confused with the three natures of Oneness, where each force is a Divine aspect. We see this in the Christian Trinity where the three are all perfect and are not active, passive, or neutral but beyond the duality of life that contains "good and evil" that can only be seen clearly in oneself, once neutrality is understood as a place of meeting the hope of Wholeness and feeling oneself without the contrast between the three forces of active, passive, and neutral.

Neutrality is the place of rest, repose, and recovery ... it is homeostatic ... transparent to the seer, so one never feels like the doer or the seer ... one never feels "seen" ... but rather one feels created as an event on the screen of life, painted by the silent hand of compassion ... one feels made with every other movement in the landscape of the moment, nothing being intrinsically good or evil.

Everything moves with ease, even in the suffering and the lesion, because the neutrality is not positioned in either.

Neutral is so different in a child than in an adult that one may miss it, literally not feel it ... I called it the "Desert Neutral" after the great teachers, who took to the desert to become whole and internally rarefied in their neutrality, i.e., in their transparency to love.

Neutral with indwelling neutrality is suffused with Third Level Stillness.

This is a Meeting Place of all incarnate life.

Therapeutics pass into the neutral substance, and a mystery unfolds as the breath of Divine love cascades, as a therapeutic force, across a night desert landscape, filling and leaving behind no visible effects ... only the emptiness of holy Stillness ... healing the physician's sense of limits ... leaving one aware of one's blindness and coarseness ... suffused.

This practical is hard to do on adults, but let's try to learn more about neutrality and the gift of it.

Neutral is the ebb ... where motions subside before a new beginning appears.

Neutral is not a means to an end ... it is the end itself.

PEDIATRICS PHASE TWO: OVERVIEW

The teachings we are presenting on the Biodynamics of Osteopathy and the treatment of children are not about techniques. We are presenting a curriculum that is part of a long legacy that has been nurtured since Dr. Still's original teaching. These teachings are little branches upon the tree of osteopathy. The tree feeds us all. The substance of the tree supports us; it is the principles that we build our thinking upon. These principles must be understood with our hands, so that the truths become a living reality, not just words.

The patient is Wholeness.

Nowhere does the above principle expose itself so easily as in the science of the osteopathic treatment of children.

We know that the growth and development of a child is a movement of Wholeness; the Whole is unfolding as a single being.

What makes a child "on time" to meet the milestones of growth and development?

Dr. Still drew us a picture of this, as did Dr. Sutherland. Their foundational view of normal was not based on anything other than what their hands reported about this Wholeness. Dr. Still often commented that osteopathy is not in a book. Then where is it?

It is an art ... a perceptual skill ... of what? ... Of understanding normal ... what is normal? ... Certainly not lesions. We are called to see more than abnormal ... we are called to something much more important. We are called to see normal.

Why would Dr. Still say that our skill comes from understanding normal?

In the first edition of Magoun's *Osteopathy in the Cranial Field,* WGS opens with a picture of normal, both his and Dr. Still's. Dr. Still describes a "supreme intelligence moving into the cerebral spinal fluid and flowing to every cell." This movement occurs without systems. It moves as if the Whole was transparent to its presence.

Visualize yourself as an empty house void of any systems, and see if you can feel the movement of creation coming in and flowing to every cell as one place ... as a whole.

As we discussed last time ... there are three levels of Stillness leading to this room. In the room we are met; then, in a flash, we change ... here we begin Phase Two of the treatment of children, and we begin with Wholeness as a theme.

We will find the room and wait. We will see Zone A, Zone B, and the Health in their wholeness as separate units of function ... then we will try to see the essential normality we spoke about ... see the movement of creation in a transparent system.

What touches us?

What is it that strikes us so completely that our higher self awakens, empty of time and identity? Beauty is Wholeness.

Dr. Still wrote:

"Solemnity takes possession of the mind, ... a smile of love runs over the face, ... the ebb and tide of the great ocean of reason, whose depths have never been fathomed, swell to your surging brain ... you eat and drink, and as you stand in silent amazement, ... suns appear where you never saw a star, brilliant with the rays of God's wisdom, as displayed in man and the laws of life, ... eternal in days, ... and as true as the mind of God himself."

Autobiography of Andrew T. Still (1897)

DIRECT AND INDIRECT METHODS IN THE TREATMENT OF CHILDREN

Historically, osteopathy in the cranial field was taught in courses designed by Harold Magoun. This was after Sutherland's death. It was well known by his closest colleagues that Will Sutherland preferred the indirect method. You can validate this by reading Lippincott's *A Manual of Cranial Technique*. I was trained by four of Sutherland's colleagues, who were in his personal study group from 1936 to 1953. He was clear about the fact that the indirect method was his choice.

Indirect methodology means "to use the motion in the lesion, and not match the forces, or use any barrier." This is rare, because most of today's teachers were influenced by Magoun, who organized and controlled the Sutherland Cranial Teaching Foundation.

Indirect methodology is safe and effective. It requires a different sense of what a lesion is. It requires one to see the motion as the lesion. That's how it's named, by its motion. This restricted motion is easily abandoned for the inertia in the lesion. The direct action mindset is that the patient's symptoms are from a cranial entrapment neuropathy. The Fluid Body dynamics of growth and development do not support this orthopedic view of osteopathy.

Biodynamic methodology is indirect, or functional, and uses the motion present in the lesion field. This means that no motion testing is necessary, only synchronization with the involuntary motion that's present.

Most commonly, we work with the Fluid Body rather than tissue because the Fluid Body is the sole force behind healing and growth.

Tissue is dynamically fluid when it is Idling or Neutral. This, of course, proves the principle that we are dealing with a fluid like protoplasm that forms all our functions, not just a watery substance.

Please take the time to think about the physiological basis of growth and healing. Please reread pages 16–17 in *Philosophy of Osteopathy.*

You cannot feel fascial planes in infants. They feel like a warm gel. Lesions only occur in the Whole. This is a fact, not a theory. This principle of Wholeness is totally accessible through the Biodynamic Method.

It is the goal of the pediatrics program that you see these realities and come to know them as "ease." The growth of a child is not a tissue war. It is a "ballet in the whole" with a theoretical tension of 2 millimeters or less of pressure.

This minimal tension is a balance point. It's all the tension necessary to unfold a complete life.

Nature does not look for lesions and manipulate them. Nature looks only for balance.

ZONE B AND THE THREE LEVELS OF STILLNESS

The ability to communicate and cooperate with the natural laws that frame the substance and activity of Zone B can lead to many wonderful clinical results.

Diagnostics in children often depend on seeing the relationship of Zone B to Zone A.

The normal Zone A (soma) is transparent to the Health and does not reflect anatomy any more than a muscle in Neutral does. As you know, a muscle in Neutral feels like a bag of water.

Let's continue with this point of seeing Zone A and Zone B and their relationship. Can you draw the picture of Zone A and Zone B in this patient?

In the first chapter of *Philosophy of Osteopathy* by A. T. Still, D.O., he asks "What is anatomy?" His reply needs your review, so you can see further than just the gross structure and understand our work in relation to the tradition that Still began. Anatomy is a living Wholeness of function and should be seen as a mystery of form, not a static, academic structure.

Additionally, my oldest osteopathic friend, Eliott Blackman, came by one summer and told me a story about Wholeness, Zone B, and osteopathy. The story is this: When in Kirksville in 1966 (Eliott's second year) he went to see Dr. Korr, our physiology teacher and author of *The Physiological Basis of Osteopathic Medicine.* He asked Dr. Korr, "Is the body a syncytium?" The answer came, "A visible segment is a segment in trouble," ...

A syncytium is a group of cells acting as a single mass of protoplasm. In the Fluid Body there is no anatomy, no somatic segments, just protoplasm. When Zone B lesions, it becomes visible as Zone A. Zone A transmutes under the influence of the Tide into Zone B.

As you evaluate your patient today, there will be a Zone A and a Zone B, but can you feel B without A? This skill is necessary.

As you find Zone B, can you feel its Wholeness? It functions as one drop. There is no distance within its mind. As you sit where you are, everything is in your hands (literally).

Once the above is clear, we are going to explore the different levels of Stillness and the landscapes in between.

The first level of Stillness is the balance point between atmospheric pressure and the fluids in the body. We find this by sensing the air in the room and the same Tide in the patient. There is not a point of interface; it is a continuum. The Stillness is a place of balance. It's calm. It's not a true stillness because it doesn't have any therapeutic potency.

Before we come to Level Two Stillness, we pass through the space of the body chemistry where we can read molecular disturbances. See what comes to you as you pass from the Level One Stillness into the breathing of the Fluid Body at 2 cpm. It may feel odd. If you work at this, you can read a variety of chemical states.

Level Two Stillness is the fulcrum for the breathing, both primary and secondary. Let's begin by asking the question, "Does the Fluid Body in this patient respond to Thoracic Respiration?" In children and saints, the Fluid Body is suffused and powered by Thoracic and Primary Respiration as one transmutative force. After checking Thoracic Respiration, you should check for Primary Respiration and its influence on the Fluid Body. Next, see if the two respirations are relating to each other or if they are strangers.

Now we move to Level Two Stillness. We sense the Stillness from which and to which the breathing comes and goes. As we wait, the Stillness moves into the foreground and Zone D comes into our awareness, automatically.

At this level, we find the Long-Tide, an ocean breathing (Zone D). Sense the ocean without any Zone A—the "house under the sea," with all the doors and windows open.

We study the next level of stillness in Phase Four, the Dynamic Stillness or Third Level Stillness. This is also "the Meeting Place."

To witness this, one must go to the fulcrum for the Long-Tide.

As we come to the effort, we enter a void. The void in the context we are using is a place where we can perceive nothing but our own limits ... it is not pleasant. But if you have worked on this, the void is no longer a void, a place of tension as the ego dissolves, but a peaceful room in the house under the sea ... a waiting place where the Tide ripens our consciousness.

As our senses are converted by the presence in the house ... we begin to see the Health ... the beauty and the transparency that we see in children.

Through this transparency comes a "wind" ... Divine and Holy ... As we are touched by this Stillness, we become aware of our own healing ... it has many dimensions, but it "holds us so completely" that we are renewed, purified, and able to move with the companionship of the host of the house ... the teacher has come ... as this awareness enters us, the whole world is seen as health ...

The movement of the creation of eternity fills our abandoning vessel as a fourth level of Stillness. The Stillness of angelic proportions. The Stillness which heralds the beginning of the return of the senses to the original state, as an expression of the Health.

THE PELVIC BOWL AND THE PERINATAL PERIOD

The process of pregnancy is a mystery colored by many cultural beliefs. The word prenatal means "before being born."

In its wholeness, pregnancy is a community affair, shaped by the elders. In the Western world this is lost. There are some exceptions, of course, but most women today face a barren landscape of support that is taxing their inner world as they carry a child.

This work, using Biodynamic principles, will prove almost miraculous in its assistance to the work of nature during pregnancy. In my 40 years of practice as an osteopathic GP, nothing has proven osteopathy more than perinatal treatment.

In this realm, we cannot imagine the truth that lies, often unseen, throughout pregnancy. It's sad that so many parents, grandparents, elders, and physicians are totally out of touch with the beauty of the unfolding of life during this time.

Pregnancy is often treated with the same mindset as for a disease.

As practitioners, we must face this void in the culture and be humble enough to be a support system that has osteopathic thinking as its basis ...

My plea here is to trust Primary Respiration and see what happens during treatment and conversations. We cannot change the world, but we can be true to our profession and our patients, one moment at a time.

All the issues of abortion, fear of a deformed child, loss of attractiveness, family addictions, support issues, personal capacities, sexuality, sensuality, affection, myths about delivery, financial issues, self- orientation to career, breastfeeding, parenting skills, vaccination, blood tests, hospitals, and insurance often overshadow the movement of creation.

Socrates said, when asked what he did, "I am a midwife ... I help people give birth to their souls." Pregnancy, in many cases, is about the birth of being ... for a whole family as they come into a reality of love.

We all die. When a child comes "in" someone will eventually "leave" ... we must feel more than ourselves at work if the responsibility of life is to be given over to life and the ocean of palpable wisdom we call the Tide.

Pregnancy is the period before the birth when it is possible to understand that we are not here to control outcomes but to respond to the intention of the creation ... it's there as peace, neutrality, change, wholeness, and mystery that we can trust.

There is another challenge we must meet ... our thinking. Pregnancy is not a biomechanical event. The tissues are not fighting, resisting, and overcoming each other. The changes are all guided by the fluid dynamics and the Tide itself.

Often osteopaths are trained to think that the changes in form that take place are tissues being forced to yield. Thinking this way contradicts nature and leads to less than adequate treatment. The idea of a "tissue war" is as far from reality as one can get regarding the changes in the mother and child during pregnancy.

The growth of the child is not biomechanical; we know that ... and ... neither is the molding of the mother. They are in the Ocean and being shaped by it. The changes in the child/mother/ocean are not segmental, nor are they dictated by somatic activity in the vertebral column oriented to a notochordal midline.

The activity is biodynamic.

The whole changes. The faces, the chests, the abdomens, the pelvises, the viscera, the consciousness, and the persons in the family circle, even if they appear indifferent, all are changing with the child ... some are changed deeply, some not at all ... this Wholeness will be discussed more.

Treating from a biomechanical concept limits the therapeutic potential for the patient. Try to feel the child and mother as a Wholeness, under the gaze of the creation. Watch what happens when all three are seen as one Wholeness.

For example, the pelvic floor is not stretched out during labor. It happens over months, but not as a stretching. The tissue changes into a moldable jelly. In the gel-like state, a fluid in the fluid opens a new shape. You can see the space open and the form change after, just like an embryo ... same teacher, same school!

You will see that the space across the ischia changes easily during the last four months.

You will see the pelvic floor thin and circumferentially widen.

You will see the space between the tents open.

You will see the uterus and ovaries travel a great distance without a war between the tissues or visceral combat.

You will see the Long-Tide ignite labor and balance the forces of the child during labor, as it opens the doors ...

The pain and travail vary with the mother's sense of the outside presence that guides the movements ...

The mother does not push the uterus ... the Tide does.

You have all seen the force the Tide can generate ... but it also opens the space before it changes position and form ... it creates a Direction of Ease that we can learn to follow, if we wish.

Our mental orientations will be such that you will not see segments or anatomy during treatment. Why? Because the Whole is shifting its Wholeness. Tissue follows later.

THE PRENATAL PELVIS

Osteopathy can prevent many hardships for children as they enter this world.

The first line of prevention is the state of the maternal pelvis and its capacity for change. The bones, ligaments, and muscles need to transmute from muscle tissue to a gel-like state. This should be, recognizably, the last month, and progress thereafter.

Treatment during pregnancy using biodynamic principles supports the metabolic changes that allow the muscles to soften into a gel. It is quite remarkable. This is easily felt during treatment of the perineum in the last month of pregnancy. The evaluation for these changes is done as Dr. Still advises in *Philosophy of Osteopathy.* One hand is placed above the pubes on the soft parts, and one below on the soft parts of the perineum. What one feels is a gel ... not soft muscles ... this gel-like state of the muscles means that the pelvis is preparing for birthing. The gel-like state almost obliterates the fascial planes that are evident in a nonpregnant pelvis. The treatment is therefore not balanced membranous tension but balanced fluid tension.

Seeing these changes should remove some of the illusions that labor is a "mechanical war" between the uterus, the child, and the pelvis. Mother Nature knows what's coming and prepares a Direction of Ease. We need to make sure that the patient is able to express these changes of the tissues becoming fluid. If this is not occurring, then we must treat the whole Fluid Body that mediates these changes.

THE PASSAGEWAY

One expression that sums up the process of birthing is that space opens, and function moves into the space in the fluid that opens. By eight months, if one senses the fluid field of the pelvis, there will be an opening, a space shaped like a spiraling tube. It will be either left or right of center. It is the passageway prepared for the child to move along as labor begins. The child's physical position should match this space. This shape is the real birth canal, so to speak. Knowing what is happening allows one to predict the movement of the child as right occiput anterior, left occiput anterior, et cetera.

Again, we see Mother Nature being fully prepared to create an amazing process. This passageway is a space in the fluid, not a musculoskeletal positional shift. It has the shape of a tunnel from the pelvic rim to the pelvic floor. The pelvic tissues will shift afterward to follow the space and its shape (exactly the same manner in which embryonic growth and development proceed; i.e., "space opens, and function moves in").

Do not try to symmetrize the pregnant pelvis or you will inhibit this process, which is asymmetrical.

FETAL MALPOSITION, TURNING BABIES

If the pelvis is treated during pregnancy, fetal malposition is preventable. We will discuss this.

Fetal malposition is treatable without any direct action techniques, either manual or with straps. This sounds crazy. In 1982, when I began teaching how to turn babies, there were many raised eyebrows. Since then, thousands of babies have been successfully turned using this simple principle of treatment. The treatment is safe, easy to accomplish, and follows the principles of osteopathy completely. All of the babies that I am aware of, from multiple sources, were turned in the last few weeks before labor. All types of fetal malposition, from transverse lies to breech, have responded to treatment.

Three percent of the cases fail to reposition. We have followed the delivery histories on some of the "failures." In most cases, the cord was around the neck in such a manner that turning may have been traumatic for the child.

Because no force is applied, the safety of this procedure is wonderful.

Why the babies turn is a mystery of nature. We have learned a lot in twenty-five years. But the principle has not changed since its beginning in 1982. The truth of an indwelling movement toward normal is validated over and over again ... this capacity to reposition around a midline is a natural occurrence in the realms of Primary Respiration. There is plenty of science that points to repositioning as a possibility. However, our mechanistic formats resist these truths even when they're stated by experts in both embryology and osteopathy … all I can say is, try the principles and see for yourself.

A Story

In 1979 a patient came to see me. She was a pediatric nurse who had been a patient before, as had some of her family members. She was 8½ months pregnant with her second child. The baby was in a transverse lie … her first child was also transverse and had to be forcibly turned. She was distraught at the idea of another forceful procedure. "Dr. Jealous, I want you to turn my baby," she said. I was shocked at her request. "I do not know how," I said. "Yes, you do," she said. "I have seen you do many unexpected things for your patients."

I resisted her commentary and she persisted … after several go-rounds with her, I decided to center the uterus around its original midline and wait. I did nothing to the child.

I laid her on her side facing me … the fundus of the uterus was lying on the table. The cervical os was higher up … so that the uterus and the passenger were downhill from the pelvis. I knew the uterus had a midline, so I lifted the fundus until the uterus and passenger were level (as with a carpenter's level). As the pregnant uterus "leveled," the patient involuntarily rolled a little toward me. I let her come, and as she did, I followed the Direction of Ease with her. The uterus wanted to go toward the spine … so we went, without any barrier … there came a sense of centering. I waited (out of ignorance) … she then sat up … I was certain I had done nothing … at no time did I feel the uterus or passenger move … it was quiet, if anything.

She called the next day. The baby had turned during the night … she was sure that the cause was osteopathy … I was rethinking the whole event … just in case there was a principle at work that I needed to recognize … I tried turning another child, and it worked … then others tried it. The results were wonderful.

Since then, children worldwide have been turned using this technique of centering the uterus on its midline ... it is hard to believe it until you do it ... the science of osteopathy comes out of the art of osteopathy.

I became more aware of the magnitude of what we do not know and how we must always "think osteopathy" and give it a chance to show itself to us, as it did to Dr. Still.

Homework

Study the embryological development of the uterus ... just look at the pictures and see the two primordia meet ... they journey as a whole toward a destination that already exists, in an invisible matrix of perfect geometry laid down at conception ... the two halves of the uterus come together around a midline (not shown in embryology texts) and center themselves upon it ... the two become one. The cervical os is on the midline, as is the apex of the fundus ... it all seems obvious to me ... If it seems questionable to you, we can review some facts from embryologists who see the precision as perfect, as did Dr. Sutherland.

The pregnant uterus has a midline that is caused by a loss of midline orientation either by the uterus (mother), the child, or both as a singularity. I sense that the mother and child share the same midline in totality ... this central midline is not in the books.

It is an understanding developed from working with elders and my own experience using Fluid Body dynamics as a primary approach. All of it is based on Sutherland's sense of direction. It is worth pondering!

THE PERINATAL PELVIS

Practical

To understand this commentary, it is necessary to understand the principle of treatment that we have gleaned from our study of cranial osteopathy and embryology.

The observations from Sutherland relative to fluid dynamics clearly focused on the intelligence, precision, and transmutative power of Primary Respiration. Together with his observations and those of many embryologists, we enter a world of principles that are very different from a biomechanical, or tissue-oriented, osteopathic principle of treatment.

The engagement of the Direction of Ease in the Fluid Body, rather than using direct or indirect action on the tissues, unveils new horizons in both healing and diagnosis.

As a foundational principle, try to imagine protoplasm (not water) at conception ... as a neutral substance that can hold an image. We call it the blueprint of life (both form and function co-emerge) ... From this comes a being (embryo) ... It unfolds (growth) ... perfectly ... and is modified by genetic confrontation.

When a being becomes sick or injured, the same forces that form the embryo are activated to repair the displacement of the whole ... this is accomplished by creating a Neutral state in the lesion field and then remolding the function to the original blueprint and its midline (one that precedes the notochord).

The Fluid Body is more intelligent than the brain, which it forms.

When our treatment uses the Fluid Body, we do not engage the nervous system as a therapeutic force, as we do when engaging tissue, as the doorway to healing.

When the Fluid Body repositions tissue, it activates a process that takes a few days ... because the treatment reorients the whole, not just the part ... Because of this holistic healing process, many symptoms that appear unrelated to the chief complaint will drop away, and often unexpected healing occurs far in excess of what biomechanics has proposed and demonstrated.

As we learn the new "laws of healing" related to Primary Respiration, we will slowly see how to interpret the Fluid Body activities ... until then, ask questions of the mentors.

All of these activities, in utero, in children, and in adults, are called Primary Respiration. The original writing in the first chapter of the first edition of *Osteopathy in the Cranial Field* needs your attention.

PRACTICAL APPLICATIONS

(First Three Levels)

Have the patient sit on your hands so that the lateral border of the ischia are touching the tip of the longest finger ...

Sense the space between the ischia to predict the adequacy of the pelvis for the passage of the child ... remember this diameter because, as pregnancy progresses, the space should change.

Sense the tissue tone of the pelvic diaphragm ... as pregnancy enters the eighth month, these tissues should be gel-like ... they should not feel like tissue ... this transmutation of the tissue to a gel is a process related to hormones and the Fluid Body ... if this is not happening, the treatment, as we will describe it, should help this change occur ... it is impressive to see how Mother Nature is getting ready for birthing ...

Sense an area circumscribed by the coccyx, the ischia, and the pubic symbiosis ... this area can be likened to a circle. The circle can be moved in a clockwise or counterclockwise manner to find tissue barriers and tissue Direction of Ease ... Sutherland taught this and used the Direction of Ease to engage a treatment ... what happens if you go in the Direction of Ease and continue without engaging a barrier?

Remember what happened ...

Now switch.

Balance fluid tension and the maternal pelvis

A pelvic bowl of protoplasm

A central Stillness that has the shape of a midline in the fluid

What transpires?

Also, read *Philosophy of Osteopathy* by A. T. Still, the chapter on obstetrics (the balancing of the soft parts above and below the pubes).

THE PERINATAL PELVIS, PART TWO

Pregnancy Should Not Be Managed as a Disease.

In many cultures there is a drama around pregnancy that is fear-based. People want to "not have any changes" in their life from the pregnancy... have a baby, no pain, and return to being the same person or couple as before. This is epidemically true. People want children without having them change their personal goals and habits. This can become a problem in many ways. The fears cause excessive testing and medication and are not dealt with to develop comfort and peace, but rather to treat pregnancy as a disease. Often there is a rush to return to work postpartum, along with a choice not to breastfeed and to take more medications to stop lactation. All of these things do affect the child. Modern medical texts sometimes even claim that formula is better than breast milk! Pregnancy is a natural wonder, and time spent with mother nature is refreshing and synchronizing. It helps to bond the mother to the "Tides" she will meet as the event ripens.

The Mother and Child Share a Midline.

We spoke about this in the first course. Turning babies depends on this knowledge.

During the last month, the tissues in the pelvis become like a gel.

This change is obvious to skilled hands. The tissue melts away into a gel-like substance that can express incredible elasticity. The pelvic floor shows this change at least three weeks before labor. Here again, we see a precognitive intelligence at work. It is an expression of the Fluid Body with the same precision we see in treatment. This is one reason we pay attention to the Fluid Body so closely during pregnancy.

During the Last Month a "Birth Canal" Appears.

We usually think of the birth canal as an anatomical passageway in the mother's tissues. Well, take another look and see if you cannot feel a shape in the Fluid Body weeks before the child engages or labor ensues. As you hold the pelvis like a bowl of water, rather than an anatomical place you will feel a curved shape on the left or right side of the pelvic bowl. This is the space opening to ease the passage of the child ... apparently the baby senses this and follows this passage as a Direction of Ease during birth.

Again ... precognition on the part of the Fluid Body. This LOA or ROA passage can be predicted by observing this.

The Ignition for Labor Comes from the Long-Tide.

When I discovered this, I was awed but not surprised. The sea around us is a potent and intelligent presence. All native cultures respect this wisdom. Sutherland was sure of it. Blechschmidt points to it indirectly. The Long-Tide comes from the horizon and enters the pelvis ... As it does, there is great fire and serenity...the uterus gets fire and Neutral ... a week or more before labor. Some mothers feel this and some have a little "false labor."

This can be felt if the mother is spiritually aware or has been given meditations on the Long-Tide ... it is a normal relationship with nature, and having it can give a mother great confidence.

The Mother and Child Can Communicate Telepathically During Labor.

Here again is more Direction of Ease for the participants ... knowing "how the child is doing" is reassuring.

Here is a perfect example of the often-repeated osteopathic principle "We are to learn how to communicate and cooperate with natural laws ... not those framed by human hands."

Dr. Still meant every word. He lived this, as did my precious teachers, who strived not to impose force upon the mind already at work, for the patient and the physician within.

With openness we can learn these ways, even though the culture at large is divorced from the "hand that feeds it."

Sutherland, in 1948, saw his relationship with the Tide very clearly, this after 50 years of effort. What persistent love must have fired his heart.

The little bit we know is enough to begin to "try and trust" the Tide ... how? By pretending the principles work. Apply them with confidence in the legacy that brought us here. As Sutherland said, the results are "uncanny." When your patients prove osteopathy to you, you will begin to believe it.

We discussed the postpartum treatment of the important seams in the first pediatrics course. The postpartum pelvis is treated with the same principles as the prenatal pelvis.

THE PELVIS

Practical

The patients sit as they did in the indirect approach.

The hands are positioned the same as before.

No tissue forces are addressed ... they should be a gel for several more weeks.

Sense only Zone B.

Wait ... at the Meeting Place of Third Level Stillness.

When your senses are transmuted, you will see or feel the midline through the pelvis ... wait.

A therapeutic event of large sweeping waves will occur ...

Do not follow closely.

At the end point there will be the sense that Thoracic Respiration is passing through the pelvis.

Amen.

MEDITATION

This meditation is real. It will help you a great deal to see a shift in yourself.

Sit in an ordinary manner, next to a child or an adult. Be relaxed, not fixed.
Sense the person next to you.
Sense the sea around you both,
everything.
Now, place all of your attention on
the sea.
What transpires?
Usually, one feels the transparency of the person and the sea
passing through.
This is the Meeting Place and it will center you.

You Should Not Treat a Child as an Adult, But You Should Treat an Adult as a Child

The Sicker the Child, the Easier the Treatment

What Is the Child Looking At in You?

THE DESERT NEUTRAL

All of these exist as "places" in the Wholeness of a child.

1. Health ... the embryonic blueprint
2. Transmutation ... the forces of death and renewal
3. Love ... the movement of creation in eternity
4. Neutral ... the point of nothingness

Each one has definite characteristics that help us to appreciate them and begin to understand the landscape of healing in children.

The Health is eternity incarnate, transparent to love, with a central identity in the movement of Wholeness. The Mystery of Health is its unerring wisdom, in both design and intention. It feels like something growing inside the child, in swirling precision.

Transmutation is the change of one thing into another, without the process of transformation ... an immediate change of being. The whole landscape shifts. This is a therapeutic force.

The love is Divine. A breath that touches and ends all separation, passing through everything as if transparent. The "I" that is everything as Self.

Neutral is a point of willingness where the forces of the Breath of Life enter for specific intention, shrouded by a veil of sanctity, a Meeting Place for unfoldment and healing. In the treatment of children, the awareness of this "place" is vital to a full therapeutic potency. This Neutral in children is always there, even in shattered systems. This place of Neutral feels like a desert ... empty and barren except for a sense of twilight and bareness. It feels like a night desert with only starlight. A place of bareness, not a void ... there is a sensation of desert and place.

The child has no self-image or self-centeredness ... the child is transparent to the Divine presence without editing.

The empty Desert Neutral is barren of intention or will ... because of this, the Desert Neutral feels very different from a Dynamic Stillness Neutral in adults, which is dark and thick and less rarefied, because adults have "observers" that thicken the Neutral that feels like a dark thick stillness ... unlike the thin emptiness of a desert surface ...

Coming to this distinct "place" and understanding that it is a Meeting Place in the child, a specific activity of being for the child, coming here helps us "see," and as we "see the seer seeing" ... we transmute and are carried into an awareness that synchronizes us into the Wholeness, and a treatment transpires. This Neutral is beyond most of us, and so it feels "odd" ... but we are adults.

When therapeutic forces enter, it feels like we are falling. The air fills and the therapeutics end. As the therapeutic force retreats, it seems to go "far away" past the stars, beyond the adult range of perception.

REVIEW OF TREATMENT OF CHILDREN

You cannot treat a child as an adult.

The science of growth and development based on embryological facts and the lineage of osteopathy established by Still, Sutherland, and their students leads to a common landscape.

Healing is guided by the fluid fields in a biodynamic system under the guidance of the presence of Primary Respiration ... this includes repositioning of form. Positioning is a non-anatomical event that flourishes under the influence of midline/fluid dynamics expressing the design of wisdom through a neutral field of unconditional potential.

The self we seek is in the "other," which, when met, suffuses our consciousness with Wholeness, eternally incarnate, located not in ourselves but everywhere. Children unveil the mystery of things that the mind and heart cannot meet. It is possible to understand children, to learn how to respond to their "world" and reawaken ours.

NEUTRAL

Practical

Synchronization, not with the breathing of Primary Respiration as we see it in adults (kids do not have rates) … but with something beautiful to you … opens you to that beauty … then the effect of that beauty changes your awareness … and a new landscape appears.

The Neutral in children is less dense than the Dynamic Stillness in adults … a more rarefied, softer, grayish silver.

This Neutral field is transparent to the "heavens" and the "stars" … when we see the Neutral field, we also see that it is an expression of something "beyond" … a place, however unseen by adults, that one knows is a Mystery. The child fills with a streaming of grace from heaven and unfolds into further growth and healing.

It is never the same twice … the format is unique to the circumstances … the treatment is crafted by a knowledge of the child's needs that leaves one humble and awake to one's limits … this is not disturbing because, as it happens, there is Third Level Stillness that feels so refreshing that one chooses health and its mystery.

Synchronization
Conversion of the senses
New landscape
Rarefied Neutral
Transparency
Space … heavenly
Connection between the child and the space above
Filling

Third Level Stillness as a place of being
A child's gaze ...

COMMUNICATION

When we arrive at this Neutral field, a form of communication begins with the newborn, infant, or child ... Many stories pass between us ... stories that cling to eternity and common sense ... stories from the language of oneness that precedes cultural language ... This is a relief for the child ... it de-stresses their curiosity about their environment, which often tries to educate the child away from Wholeness into a cultural similarity ... Language in a child is looked upon as "undeveloped" when in fact there is a first language, and we can recover a lot of ourselves by learning it from children ... This is another reason why the Desert Neutral is so meaningful ... it is the center of the unfoldment, of incarnation (growth and development), as well as adaptation to the stress of this "world," as presented to children by "grown-ups."

Also, the sense of "me" here and "you" there that has infected the observer in adults is not present in children ... children cannot heal if all their energy is engaged in adaptation to a "negative" environment, rather than healing in an environment that "sees" them as they are and meets them on their ground ... emptiness, barren of self-image ... a place of Desert Neutral ... where we all meet, without the memory of time and circumstance.

Children cannot be treated as adults. We are adults ... we need their help to "see" them as they are ... When we see them seeing through us into a desert place in us ... we begin to remember eternity and become, for a second, like a child ... They, as we all know, awaken our real self.

We can treat from this place in ourselves and learn the principles set forth by the Tide ... principles rarely seen in adults because of the overlay of self-image … we are all learning new things by treating this way … it is humbling and rich and challenging …

REMOLDING THE CHILD

Birth is a CV4 followed by an EV4.

The forces of labor exceed 100 psi.

Why does the child not rupture?

100 psi on any tissue surface in a newborn would do incredible damage.

The tissue would tear apart under this kind of force. I believe that the Fluid Body and the fluid in the fluid (potency) are able to withstand these pressures much more easily than the tissue. We are trained to think that the tissue is balancing the stress, but think about another force as well... that of the collective potency of Primary Respiration as well as just plain hydraulics.

Once birthed, the head and body remold into the blueprint of the Health. How? It is known to be Fluid Body activity. We know this, and yet we are insisting on moving the bones, directly.

Remolding is accomplished in 72 hours, maximum. A caput succedaneum may take a little longer.

If the Neutral is not obtained, then the remolding is delayed, and one should suspect a problem with the Fluid Body if remolding is delayed even one day.

Any deformity needs two basic activities to heal: the Fluid Body integrity and Neutral in the Whole. Fluid body integrity means fluid drive (power to do work), ignition, a relationship with the true midline, elasticity (six directions), and Neutral dynamics.

In our first course, we studied how to help the Fluid Body heal by association with the indwelling Stillness. Now we will continue that study in a little more detail.

DOORWAY BETWEEN ZONE B AND THE OCEAN

Practical

Draw the Fluid Body and its false midline.

Now assess:

The opacity

The fluid drive

The fire

The elasticity ... all six directions of disengagement

Capacity for Neutral

Treat using the doorway between Zone B and the ocean.

What is the end point, as it occurred in your patient?

CHILDREN'S SENSORIUM

Children live in a sensorium that is way beyond ours.

However, we can at times sense the infinity of that distance and wait as the therapeutic substance comes down into and fills the child ... more is written on this, i.e., the Desert Neutral, which is about the unique nature of Neutral in infants.

The last practical explored the orderliness of life and the landscapes that we pass into as we follow the path left by WGS. The tool he gave us, "where's the fulcrum," is not, as you know, a lesson in physics, but a search for the cause of the individual landscapes ... each one the unfolding of a branch of creation.

Synchronization is about beauty...

But now we begin to see that there is a third level of Stillness that is the ground level of life in the "house under the sea" ... children feel at home here ...

For us, this Third Level Stillness can be remembered ... and as such, it becomes our Zone C ... synchronization then comes to us from the child that breaks the spell of self-centering and converts our senses, so we see a Wholeness of love and suffering ... suffused with the hand of compassion.

From this comes transparency, and another type of therapeutic fire (potency).

We explored chemistry, breathing, doorways, and efficiency ... each level unique in spatial dynamics and tempo.

Now we explore breathing, Zone B, and Third Level Stillness as a potential Wholeness ... a child breathes as a Whole ... Zones B and A form a singular response to creation ... Thoracic Respiration and Primary Respiration co-emerge as one function ...

Thoracic respiration is as potent as a Tide, as is Primary Respiration with no rate ... they suffuse each other ...

As we work on ourselves, we will notice our Thoracic Respiration and Zone B ... see what transpires!

Then a practical noticing of diagnostics for A and B ... then using Third Level Stillness to engage a therapeutic process ... in B.

Later we will see fire ...

MEDITATION

The Breathing in Children Is Not Like That in an Adult

The observation of our own breathing can help us understand children. Our Thoracic Respiration and primary respiratory rate obliterate the simple breath that is united and holy in us.

This simple breath is related to the Health, as it is in us.

As we watch our breathing, we can move into the Meeting Place ... a Third Level Stillness in the sea around us and through us. Here is where we are met by the eternal in various "forms" ... the master of the house, the embryonic breath, the breathlessness that precedes the meeting.

In Pediatrics One, there was feedback that as we settled into this Meeting Place there was "fear." What is fear? What changes it?

Fear is the central fulcrum of the ego (in the Western sense) ... As we descend into the darkness of the subconscious, the senses have less and less stimulation ... until they have none.

Here is where the fear enters as well, as a variety of unpleasant thoughts and emotions. This is the content of your subconscious. It is always there and is now unveiled ... in our culture we are constantly craving stimulation for gratification of the ego. Now that we have no stimulation, all hell breaks loose trying to capture material meaning. The ego develops in our brain as synapses ... now they continue to fire, even when not beckoned ... one discovers that one is not free. That freedom lies in the capacity for Neutral and the freedom to choose which event to enter or not enter. This is the basis of *The Divine Comedy* by Dante.

This fear will end once we see it as "not me" ... even though we are sometimes in it and choosing it. This is not the Health, not one's higher self, not the Christ within; it is simple "fear" ... of losing one's identity, as built by the ego, in the brain synapse of childhood.

When the observer sees that this fear is not the Health ... then the observer deepens, and one can rest at the Meeting Place. Ask yourself, when you are ready, whether we can, as adults, love as children do ... and why is that, why?

As we see the breathing ... we move deeper into ease ... and Neutral.

Then we come to a quiet place and wait.

Then we are transmuted, and we awaken to a new landscape.

Can you notice the moment when you are transmuted into a new person?

There are several books that can help:

Into the Silent Land, Martin Laird
News Seeds of Contemplation, Thomas Merton
Zen Mind, Beginner's Mind, Shunryu Suzuki
A Testament of Devotion, Thomas Kelly
The Collected Works of St. John of the Cross

A MEDITATION FOR PRENATAL WOMEN

Go outside and listen, as far away as you can.

The air around us is fluid; there is a movement that passes through that fluid slowly.

Lie down, look at the tree overhead ... then observe the space between the branches and leaves, and wait.

Maybe your pregnant patients can connect with nature this way and be more aware of the Wholeness of birthing.

QUOTES FROM SEVEN- TO NINE-YEAR-OLD CHILDREN

In 1979, a dance teacher from New York, who summered in rural Maine, told me that during her treatments she could feel the warm fluid movements. This occurred on a regular basis after she had her first three treatments. She taught children to dance and express fluidity in motion. She wondered if children could naturally feel what we called Primary Respiration.

She set up an experiment. She asked the children to feel inside themselves and report … nothing more was said.

The results are as follows:

"It felt like a sea of many people that were fighting over me."

(Joanna, grade 3)

"My imagination works with the whole body and looks like crawling on grass."

(Jason, grade 4)

"Mine looks like a brain, feels like a big circle in my head."

(JoAnn, grade 2)

“My imagination is like a blob. It changes shape, size and color. If you could feel it, it would feel slippery and spongy. It scoops up ideas and squeezes them into one idea. It fixes it up so that it is as good as can be and sends it to my mind. My mind sends it to my hands, and I do it.”

(Alan, grade 4)

“It felt like someone was in a boat. It felt like I was in a boat.”

(Daniel, grade 3)

“My imagination changes by the minute. Now it’s in my stomach.”

(Jacob, grade 2)

“Opening and closing.”

(Ryan, grade 2)

“My mind has many thoughts. Today her thought is a bird. Not just any bird though!”

(Erin, grade 4)

“Blue fire, fierce fire.”

(Dale, grade 4)

"I can't go inside my mind without going side to side. It's so windy. I find out that the wind is wavy, and it has special vitamins to pick up things."

(Renee, grade 3)

"If it is trapped, it feels like it is going to die."

(Amy, grade 4)

"Wee-hee-hee-hee-hee-hee."

(Keith, grade 4)

"It wants to be free. It doesn't want to be in an enclosed area. It likes to just be a nice summer breeze."

(Jennifer, grade 4)

"Freedom!"

(Nicholas, grade 4)

"Very very wavy."

(Angela, grade 4)

"It feels like there is a bunch of water in my head, spinning around. It feels like firemen are spraying water in my head."

(JB, age 7)

If children can feel the "Fluid Body" and observe it, then we must be careful to realize and honor their sensibilities and natural gifts. Children are invaded by many good intentions ... therefore, education of ourselves and the parents is important.

KEY POINTS

Children should not be treated as adults.

Let the Health in the child center you.

Children do not have rates unless one is induced by the operator.

Children do not have either static anatomy or parts.

Wholeness is a reality that must be met without compromise.

Seeing the natural therapeutic dynamics of Wholeness in a child, rather than rearranging the parts, can only be done if one is centered by the child.

Erich Blechschmidt, a noted embryologist, states that the process of growth and development is a mystery known only to the embryo; this means it is knowable, but only from certain states of being.

The transparency of a child radiates a mystery of love and beauty.

The Health that we all wish to see is wholly seen when we see it seeing us.

Eternity passes into our temporal mind and re-centers us in the Health.

The beauty we see, even in the gravest of suffering, is the place where one can see the motion of the mystery we call therapeutics.

Learning to be "centered by the Health" of the child is like looking into the eyes of a great and beautiful love ... the child, no manner what degree of suffering it experiences, is transparent to its true nature ... Adults lose their capacity to feel Divine love and focus on getting away from their lesions ... but a child's being is a dwelling place where love and suffering suffuse each other, leaving the child's presence unalterable, even if physically there are severe deformities ... this presence is the power that will center you.

The mind must be neutral ... not active, wanting to know ... not passive, wanting to surrender ... but neutral, not wanting or waiting ... empty of any goal, even that of Neutral ... remember protoplasm in neutral ... idle ... substantial without format ... then something enters.

Being Neutral is unnatural for an educated mind, or for anyone with a need to have control.

A child's gaze comes through them, not from them ... as it enters the emptiness of your Neutral mind ... there will be a depth touched in you that feels like the bottom of a deep well ... this place is what we call the Meeting Place ... once the meeting occurs ... it is followed by a sense of new being. Hold onto this all through treatment ... why hold onto it? ... Because your old habits will cloud it over ... Later, it will come easier and require less discipline to stay with the beauty and "new mind," which is your health.

Let's go to work and then we will share our observations on the "observer" and "observers" in ourselves ... remember, we are studying the Neutral mind and the effect of the child's health on us.

BREATHING IN CHILDREN AND ADULTS

Our sense of breathing, as a function in the cranial field of osteopathy, has always been that there are three basic breaths: Thoracic or Secondary Respiration, Primary Respiration, and the Breath of Life.

Thoracic respiration is a metabolic event that begins at conception and is not a mechanical, but rather a physiological, event. It is much more than the diaphragm, the lungs, and the ribs. It is intracellular metabolic fire. It heats us, and, as we shall see, it has therapeutic power. Sutherland began his journey appreciating much more about Thoracic Respiration than we commonly teach. His choice of the fourth ventricle for a CV4 was because his goal in treatment was to bring the motion of Thoracic Respiration to a highly refined Neutral, where the breathing was almost still. He saw this Neutral of Thoracic Respiration as a primary indicator that the fluids, especially the lymphatics, were free to find homeostasis. Rereading his comments is inspiring. In children, we have discovered that Thoracic Respiration has transmutative therapeutic potency, something we will explore over the next year.

Primary respiration is hallmarked by an inhalation period and an exhalation period (Sutherland). Primary respiration has a variety of rates. The common rates are two to three cycles per minute and 100 seconds per cycle.

In the two-to-three-cycle-per-minute rate, the period of inhalation and the period of exhalation each last 12 seconds ... the whole cycle being 24 seconds, or two and a half cycles per minute.

The rate of the Long-Tide is 50 seconds per exhalation period and 50 seconds for the inhalation period, the whole cycle being 100 seconds (Becker).

The cranial rhythmic impulse of the Long-Tide is not considered a rate, because it is the same as Thoracic Respiration and is highly variable ... it is considered by many to be a nontherapeutic rate. This view is not appreciated by everyone and needs your personal exploration as to its validity.

As you may recall, during therapeutics in adults, the inhalation phase is prolonged and the exhalation phase is silent. This phenomenon demonstrates that rates are not present while transmutation is occurring, and that when the treatment period is ending, there comes a Stillpoint that heralds a new Neutral, which is coming. The Stillpoint is the height of the transmutative period and is followed by a Neutral at a deeper level than the beginning Neutral. The rate also slows, so that the initial Neutral is often breathing faster than the Neutral at the end point, after transmutation occurs.

This change to a slower rate indicates a greater Wholeness, a deeper Neutral that is more stable and with greater therapeutic outcomes.

Eventually, we come to a Neutral with no rate ... just a steady Dynamic Stillness that hovers in the fluid indefinitely. This is Primary Respiration, but the breathing of inhalation and exhalation has become "breathless and still" ... not as in Stillpoint, but as a state of being that persists.

So ... we have many levels of Neutral that can appear in relation to what we call Primary Respiration ... each one with a unique landscape of temporal and spatial dynamics.

Adults consistently demonstrate separate fulcrums for Thoracic Respiration, Primary Respiration, and the Breath of Life. We have therefore assumed that this is true for children. We also see that the potency to transmute is exclusive to the power of Primary Respiration in adults. We do not see a potency that can transmute connected to Thoracic Respiration in adults. And the Breath of Life rarely consumes the adult patient in a miraculous healing that defies natural laws, as we have theorized them in our profession.

Children do not follow the adult framework ... the uniqueness of their primary respiratory dynamics causes us to pause as we begin to witness the abyss between being a child and being an adult. We are learning to rethink what we know and letting our neutrality guide us further, using our ignorance as a means of becoming consistently Neutral and free to observe "laws not framed by human hands" (A. T. Still).

CHILDREN AND PRIMARY RESPIRATORY DYNAMICS

Once our perception is "centered by the Tide" ... the world looks very different than it does "under our own power" ... the quote we read from Dr. Still reflects his most intimate inner life. His perception was shifted, and as he said, "There are suns where you never saw a star."

The Tide heals our patients but also heals us. The dross falls away. The scales that veil our eyes are removed, and our senses begin to move as one sense, free of slavery to our egos and all the pain and isolation therein.

As the Tide has helped us to see children more clearly, it has become apparent that there is a true Oneness and Wholeness to a healthy child. It has always fascinated me that spiritual teachers recognize the need for "seekers" to become like children ... Christ, who was always a great healer, repeatedly admonished his disciples and the rabbis to see this truth ... to become like children, so they could find heaven within them: "Verily I say unto you, Except ye be converted, and become as little children, ye shall not enter into the kingdom of heaven" (Mathew 18:3, King James Version).

Thoracic Respiration, Primary Respiration, and the Breath of Life have only one fulcrum. They share a single potency. They have different rates (sometimes), but like different leaves on one branch, they are moved as a Wholeness by the winds of creation.

Our first practical today is about reuniting the Wholeness of breathing.

When a child has surgery, very often they separate Thoracic

Respiration from the one fulcrum that it previously shared with "all the breath." The chief symptom of this is often a perceptual change in the child, one of distance ... look into their eyes, and you will see they feel "lost," separated from the Wholeness ... they become confused and "clingy."

Often a simple resynchronization of Thoracic Respiration, easily done, produces immediate and lasting perceptual shifts. In my own practice, I was missing this easy diagnosis because I assumed that Thoracic and Primary Respiration were separate functions with separate potencies and fulcrums ... this is not true in children.

Now I am wondering how many autistic and perceptually fragile children are missing this linkage, and if we are treating in a too-complex manner in some cases ... I recommend that, in your perceptually challenged children, you explore this benefit of resynchronization through the diaphragm, and see if it sorts out some of the dilemmas that we face.

THE WHOLE PATIENT

Practical

With your hands on the posterior midline of the diaphragm, synchronize with the breathing or breathlessness and watch the Whole patient ... what transpires?

Children treat faster and more easily, as adults have a split in their fulcrum. More later.

BREATHING AND CHILDREN

We have taken our understanding of Primary Respiration in adults and tried to impose that on children.

We must begin to let the normal state of a child teach us. We must start over again as a community and share our views, building a new image of what Primary Respiration is and what it means in the treatment of children.

There are two distinct breaths in children.

One is the unified expressions of Primary Respiration and Thoracic Respiration.

The other is the Breath of Life.

A wholly love-filled, self-emptying, and sweet movement that fills the child from the "stars."

When I first saw this reality, the contradiction it presented to my model of Primary Respiration was acute and unending.

I saw this oneness as a beacon of hope for everyone. In that moment the old died ... the new understanding made so much sense ...

Wholeness is the smallest part of a child.

If Primary and Thoracic Respiration are as one in children, and the Breath of Life is the "other breath" ... then what we notice is that Primary and Thoracic Respiration are created by the Breath of Life as a single potency ... they co-emerge, continually.

We also see that this single therapeutic force in children is much deeper than what is seen in adults, at least in the sick ones we treat.

If what I have seen is true ... then how is it that we see two aspects ... Thoracic Respiration with one rate of expression and Primary Respiration with another...?

First of all, oneness does not mean everything moves with the same tempo.

Second, if you watch a tree in the wind, you will see branches and leaves moving at different rates, and some not moving at all, but all on the same fulcrum, the tree—each individual motion having a small fulcrum but under the guidance of the larger tree.

The rate of Thoracic Respiration is of course variable, but observe a sleeping child to see into this reality. Transparency and holiness are evident. Sleeping children fall deeply into their Neutral.

During Neutral, normal is presenting itself to our senses. We feel awed, humbled.

In this transparency, our senses are rinsed of the dust of self-interest, and we see into the moment ... we see the long lever of the Breath of Life ... coming into the child from a place beyond the stars and beyond the gaze of an adult. The Breath of Life is restoring, igniting, and healing ... sometimes all at once ... sometimes at different moments ...

Slowly, we come to realize that children live in Neutral.

They are so different from adults that we must begin again to think osteopathically about what their normal state is.

THORACIC RESPIRATION AND PRIMARY RESPIRATION IN CHILDREN

Thoracic and Primary Respiration begin at or before conception.

They move as one branch of a tree, one fulcrum at two rates. Watch the leaves and branches of a tree in the breeze and you will see what I mean.

When children lesion, they lesion as a whole, and often this relationship, this oneness of breathing, remains. So we check for this. Hopefully it is as it should be.

If the breaths are separate, they should resynchronize as the whole of Zone B becomes Neutral. This can be appreciated easily. As the Thoracic Respiration moves into a deep inhalation (big sigh), the Primary Respiration makes a big inhalation also. This augmentation is automatic.

If this does not occur when Primary Respiration rebalances and swells, then have the child breathe in at the same moment as the Tide swells. This will resynchronize the system. If not, note this. It is important (this principle was used by WGS and is called breath augmentation). This helps Zone A and Zone B reunite as one movement in which A transmutes.

THE FIRST BREATH

The first breath of a newborn has always been a moment of marvelous beauty and relief.

In pediatrics texts there are many notable points of evaluation and remedy that one should already know.

This commentary, then, is about osteopathic vital signs related to this first breath and how it creates momentum for present and future health issues. Little is written on this subject, but the oral teaching has been passed on for decades.

Of all the courses I attended that mentioned the first breath, the person who made the most sense to me was Dr. Fulford. He focused on the long-term sequelae of those who had not completed the "first breath," those who were desynchronized during pregnancy.

Completion of the first breath creates momentum in growth/development.

The fullness of completion results in a whole individual, aligned consciously and able to function fully. These words, coming from Dr. Fulford, were few and valued. What did he mean?

My understanding, while talking to him, was based upon knowledge of the mystical path he had followed and what the words "whole," "individual," "consciously aligned," and "free-willed" would mean in sacred language.

Children are remarkably complete, whole, and free. They unfold from the blueprint of life set at conception. In order for development to unfold continuously, one must have a well-established fulcrum for Primary Respiration, Thoracic Respiration, and ignition ... in order to respond to the movement of creation as it flows through them.

At the time of first breath, the demands of life are increasing severely… the ignition creates more fire, the Long-Tide is orchestrated, the Dynamic Stillness moves in through the midline, and as the air rushes into the lungs, one breath is set in time as eternity comes ashore.

This is my understanding of the Wholeness that Dr. Fulford mentioned to me in 1979.

To be an individual, in Dr. Fulford's terminology, means to follow the destiny of unfoldment, not worldly images. The journey for Dr. Fulford was to listen to the Love behind creation and follow its voice. The result of this hard work would be to become what God made one for, not what one's genetics and ego might overlay.

The first breath establishes memory and the vital oneness that carries one's name. If the first breath is weak, our struggle to know ourselves may be extended and spiritual maturity delayed, prolonging the sense of isolation from the Divine in ourselves.

To be consciously aligned means, in the context of his work, to be aware of Divine will, to have an instinctual need to be in the presence of love and perfection.

Free will, as Dr. Fulford put it, is when one has no slavery to habits or beliefs. One is free to be shifted by the movement of the creator's hand. One is free to lighten the load of world suffering. One is detached, impartial to everything, and responsive to the unfoldment of God's love. This is not a "willy-nilly" going with the love … it is love meeting love with no preconceived outcome. It is fearlessness in the face of one's lesions.

In the Biodynamic life, the first breath is relative.

The first true breath is at or before conception. Obviously, Thoracic Respiration (O_2 metabolic exchange) begins much earlier than birth.

The presence of Primary Respiration guiding conception is a Biodynamic principle that emerges from both osteopathy and embryology.

The birthing breath is the first earthly breath, and ideally it triggers thoracic, primary, and the ignition to move together as one.

Think about the capacity of Zone B to do its work, to accomplish unfoldment of the blueprint of life, if the first breath is desynchronized and weakened.

The first hint of this, if you are not trained to see it through Fluid Body dynamics, is slowness in the remolding of the head after birth. This should be a red flag that there is a problem in the core.

At conception, the Divine image is breathed into protoplasm (clay). The perfect image is made; we call it the Health. This is a lifelong reference point for normal that is indispensable for healing and unfoldment. Without this, life does not move forward, it decays. Protoplasm is the first moldable substance that can hold an image, and the image is unerring in its timing and geometry of unfoldment. The inscription is immortal.

This could be called the absolute first breath.

Reflection on this surpasses the written history of human life.

Each of us must think about this truth in light of the clinical and personal outcomes we experience day to day in our work.

Birth

Fire, ignition, O_2, Dynamic Stillness ...
Breath of Life
The child, one breath ... incarnation unfolds.

THE WHOLENESS

Nowhere else does the above principle expose itself so easily as in the science of the osteopathic treatment of children.

We know that the growth and development of a child is a movement of Wholeness; the Whole is unfolding as a single form.

What we see in treatment are not the systems that we evaluate for milestones, which are so often used as diagnostic doorways to determine normality in children. What we see, and are interested in, is the cause of these milestones—what makes a child "on time" to meet the milestones of growth and development.

Dr. Still drew us a picture of this, as did Dr. Sutherland. Their foundational view of normal was not based on anything other than what their hands reported about this Wholeness.

Dr. Still often commented that osteopathy is not in a book. Then where is it? It is an art ... a perceptual skill ... of what? ... To understand normal ... what is normal? ... Certainly not lesions. We are called to see more than abnormal ... we are called to see something much more important. We are called to see normal. Why would Dr. Still say that our skill comes from understanding normal? What does knowing normal have to do with skill? Know normal, find the Health. What a unique basis for healing.

In the first edition of Magoun's *Osteopathy in the Cranial Field*, WGS opens with a picture of normal, both his and Dr. Still's.

Dr. Still describes a "supreme intelligence moving into the cerebral spinal fluid, and flowing to every cell, bringing order (perfect function and form)." This movement occurs without systems. It moves as if the Whole was transparent to its presence.

Visualize yourself as an empty house void of any systems, and see if you can feel the movement of creation coming in and flowing to every cell as one place ... as a Whole.

Dr. Sutherland himself goes on to make a similar commentary about the Breath of Life passing through, bringing fire (ignition) to the Whole.

These teachings of Still and Sutherland are remarkably similar to those of Dr. E. Blechschmidt as he describes a mysterious force biodynamically creating the Wholeness of growth and development, bringing form and function to every cell (biokinetics).

In the 1953 *OCA Journal,* Thomas Schooley paints another image of the same nature in his article on fulcrums. He is astoundingly clear.

In the Biodynamics of the treatment of children, we are confining ourselves to the discipline recommended by our teachers. This is difficult ... it is easier to feel lesions and make somatic engagements ... but the theory is wrong ... children do not heal by somatic or central nervous system forces. Healing is orchestrated by the same forces that cause growth and development ... the embryonic fields ... the metabolic movements of Primary Respiration ... at the most essential level, there is a Wholeness suffused by the Breath of Life, which brings order, wisdom, and existence to each being.

Wholeness, and its transparency to the Breath of Life, is all children have as therapeutics ... they do not heal in pieces. Working on pieces is popular, but working with the Wholeness is much more effective.

Being aware of Wholeness is not easy for an adult.

We must allow our senses to convert to a new landscape.

This is difficult because our intellects and egos want the stage. It could require 15 to 20 years of practice to heal this self-centered ideation in ourselves.

But!

Children awaken this in us! If we are in the right place to meet a child ... the effect of their presence on us is powerful enough to change our consciousness.

One feels this in mind and body as a kind of simple movement and openness. In Pediatrics One, we spoke about the Meeting Place, a room where we wait. It is easy to miss this place, slip back to another level of Stillness and think we are at the Meeting Place. I would warn you not to think this is a skill that will stick easily. We must see what it is that meets us and see the conversion in ourselves, directly ... as we are touched and healed in ourselves.

This great principle of osteopathy, the principle of Wholeness, is not just words for us to repeat ... to touch and be touched by Wholeness is to understand the depth of what our teachers carried in the art of osteopathy. This can be lost if we do not "practice what we preach."

As we discussed last time ... there are three levels of Stillness leading to this room; in the room we are met, then in a flash we change.

Now we begin "The Treatment of Children." We begin with Wholeness as a theme. We will find the room and wait. We will see Zone A, Zone B, and the Health in their Wholeness as separate units of function ... then we will try to see the essential normality spoken about above, and ... see the movement of creation in a transparent system. This is what is needed to help children regain the motion of growth, development, and healing. What is it that strikes us so completely that our higher self awakens, empty of time and identity?

There are many answers.

Beauty is Wholeness. Review the teaching on a normal child. Any one of these characteristics can touch and transmute an open mind. When you look past the suffering and see the Health, one of these aspects may hit your heart. Watch and wait. See yourself as you open and see a new landscape, see your body change as your mind changes, see what touches and heals you.

Let it remind of a forgotten name …
Yours!
Normal exists
Health exists
Creation i*s n*ow

Wholeness …

Dr. Blackman: "Dr. Korr, do you think a human being is a syncytium?"

Dr. Korr: "Yes, a visible segment is a segment in trouble."

Dr. Blackman: "You mean it is seamless?"

Dr. Korr: "Yes."

Kirksville, 1967

NEITHER/NOR

Beyond the dualities of our logic and refined, rational attitudes is love ... Children are special in many ways, but one that stands out very clearly during osteopathic treatment is that children are beyond any single category of definition.

They transcend the dualities that we, as adults, often insist upon without knowing. The neutrality that treatment descends into children is different than adult Neutrals ... this grayish desert-like place has no location, nor is it nowhere.

It neither breathes nor is breathless
It is neither created nor uncreated
It has neither form nor formlessness
It neither contracts nor expands
It is neither in time nor in timelessness
It is neither born nor dies
It can neither lesion nor heal
It has neither wholeness nor parts

BASICS IN THE TREATMENT OF CHILDREN

They are not adults...

Children should not be treated as adults.

Let the Health in the child center you...

Children do not have rates unless one is induced by the operator...

Children do not have either static anatomy or parts... this is a fact.

Wholeness is a reality that must be met without compromise... Still was clear on this, as is the science of embryology.

A child is a mystery, indefinable in scientific terms...

Erich Blechschmidt, a noted embryologist, says that the process of growth and development is a mystery known only to the embryo... this means it is knowable, but only in certain states of being...

Recommended reading: *Sein Und Werden* (Being and Becoming), by Erich Blechschmidt, M.D. (especially pages 89-92)

Dr. Becker, Dr. Sutherland, and Dr. Still all tried to communicate the notion that the Health can center us... they pointed toward a method of being that was not technique-driven or direct action... a review of the 1965 Sutherland memorial lecture by Dr. Becker is very descriptive.

Seeing the natural therapeutic dynamics of Wholeness in a child, rather than rearranging the parts, can only be done if one is centered by the transparency of their nature, which radiates a mystery of love and sun-like beauty.

The Health that we all wish to see is only seen when we see it seeing us and respond without thinking …

Eternity passes into our temporal mind and re-centers it on the Health. The beauty we see, even in the face of the gravest of suffering, is the thread that leads to the interface with healing … beauty descending along a path not visible to those at the bottom of the mountain.

As we work in the practicals, we are studying the art of observation that allows the treatment of children to be aligned with their needs, not the proportional orientation of adult diagnostics.

Learning to be "centered by the Health" of the child is like looking into the eyes of a great and beautiful love … the child, no matter what degree of suffering it experiences, is transparent to its true nature … Adults lose their capacity to feel Divine love and therefore focus on getting away from their lesions …

A child's being is a dwelling place where love and suffering suffuse each other, leaving the child's presence unalterable, even if physically there are severe deformities … this presence is the power that will center you.

Your mind must be neutral … not active, wanting to know … not passive, wanting to surrender or yield … but neutral, not wanting or waiting for anything … empty of any goal, even that of Neutral … remember, protoplasm is neutral and substantial. Neutral has a lovingness of unalterable tranquility.

Being Neutral is unnatural for an educated mind, or for anyone with a need to have information that fits a preconceived idea.

A child's gaze comes through them, not from them … as it enters the emptiness of your neutral mind, there will be a depth touched in you that feels like the bottom of a deep well … this place is what we call the Meeting Place … once the meeting occurs it is followed by a sense of new being … hold onto this all through treatment … why hold onto it? … Because your old habits will cloud over it … later it will come easier and require less discipline to stay with the beauty and your "new mind," which is your health and operates from information that is very different from treatment plans per se ... All this operates in a Direction of Ease ... but not for the ego ...

Let's go to work and then we will share our observations on the "observer" and "observers" in ourselves ... remember, we are studying the Neutral mind and the effect of the child's health on us.

Later, we will discuss another truth about children ... there are not individual bony osteopathic lesions.

Sense your Fluid Body and Third Level Stillness

Watchfulness

The other pair of hands is inside the child

Inside in a pool of liquid light

THE PERCEPTUAL JOURNEY TO THE MEETING PLACE

There Are Many Doorways to the Meeting Place in the House Under the Sea.

One method is as follows:

Sit. Place your hands on the patient without any technique, just the usual habit that you have.

Then dismiss the habit and wait.

A new landscape will appear.

Wait some more; the landscape will reveal its dimensionality.

Detachment (move toward love).

Wait. There will come an emptiness and then ... Neutrality ... an end in itself, not a means to "more."

Something holy enters ... there is a change in your being.

You see the location in eternity.

Go with precision and slowness.

CHILDREN AS ONE

We have spoken about many things concerning children. They are very universal and beautiful ... there is more.

Children can move the therapeutic forces in a direction that reflects great compassion flowing through them, without any spiritual training. That's correct. They can move the therapeutic power to others.

They are natural saints, bringing validation to an open heart.

As we explore their world, we come to a sense that children universally see all children as a single appendage of creation.

There is this redemptive spirit in children that allows for the treatment to go to others in need.

Redemptive prayer is practiced in most traditions. It is prayer that is done for others, like fasting for others or doing penance for others. Gandhi was well known for this kind of work.

The Wholeness of a child's heart is beyond what we can imagine.

ALL THE CHILDREN WHO WILL NEVER BE TREATED

Practical

As we work, let's open the space of the treatment to include all the children who will never be treated.

Keep it simple and see if this has any value for you.

A CHILD'S SENSE OF WHOLENESS, THE FAMILY CIRCLE

A child's experience of Wholeness is alive. For adults the memory of this has faded.

Children sense the family as one Zone B and are intent on everyone being in it. This Zone B we call the family circle. Many parents are not in it. They do not see their children as teachers. The people who honor and love the child as divine will enter the circle. It is not genetic.

When you treat a child, it helps if you respect their world. This means keeping a sense of the family Zone B in your awareness as you treat. Children feel the Health in the parents, even if the parents are dissociated from it themselves.

Children never stop loving their parents, even if thinking as adults that they have no concern for them. For a child, there is only one midline, not three or several.

Imagine your midline is not "yours." Imagine a midline where we gather as one under the mantle of creation and love. We lose our sense of being independent, alone.

If we are not aware of these things, then the child will try to heal us.

WHOLENESS

Practical

When was the last time you were aware of this Wholeness with your parents, with your children or children you love? ...

Just reflect for a moment.

Sense the family circle for the adult you are working with. Remember, it contains only those who love the person as divine.

Remember that the Third Level Stillness is the doorway.

MAINTAINING A TREATMENT

Shakedown ... peritoneal sac ... fluid to fluid in the whole.

Massage at 2 to 0 mm pressure ... long axis decompression ... toward the center of the Fluid Body.

Bathtub ... move the baby to move the water, then let the water move the baby.

Under all the breathing is breathlessness

A desert

Divine grace waters it.

THE FAMILY CIRCLE ... PERSONAL MEDITATION

Several years ago, we started working with the family circle on a personal basis. The family circle has many layers and rooms. In the center is your Health, your divine nature, perfect and transparent as a child to the movement of creation (love).

The circle is dynamic. It is a diagram you can fill out whenever you feel the need to connect with your sense of family. The family that we speak of here may or may not contain your genetic family. This is a family of friends that interface with you at different levels, some who see you in roles and identities and some who see your health rather than your persona.

Using this circle can bring you to a Meeting Place and a clarity that is supportive of your journey toward your spiritual goal.

POTENCY AND FIRE

The word "potency," as you know, means indwelling power. The word has been used in cranial work for 70 years. The sensory experience is variable depending upon which potency is present.

In children, if one feels for fire, one will meet the potency that provides the transmutation in children.

We also know that Thoracic Respiration and Primary Respiration unfold from the same fulcrum, and in a healthy child they are sharing that original fulcrum.

Thoracic respiration should be felt as fire; the movement of the physiology is fire.

Both Primary and Thoracic Respiration are fire.

Working for this realization is invaluable.

You should treat an adult as a child.

Love your neighbor as yourself.

When seen by a child
Your seer is seen
Then you sense the presence of the seer
Then the observer is transmuted … converted …
It dies in this love

BIODYNAMICS OF OSTEOPATHY BOOK SERIES

This book is one of a series of twelve *Biodynamics of Osteopathy* books. It is recommended that you read the whole series in order, as each book builds on the understanding from prior books. It is also recommended that you seek experienced teachers and mentors to help you experience the full depth of the information given.

The full series is as follows:

Phase One is about involuntary motion, which is motion present in the whole and in the lesion. We learn to synchronize with the breathing of Primary Respiration before we approach any treatment. This synchronization is the key to working with stable rates and not irritating the system. The principle of synchronizing with a healthy aspect of the patient suffuses the whole teaching program. This synchronization shifts our awareness to a different level of receptivity, which allows us to see Primary Respiration rather than the lesion field, and this eventually leads us to an understanding of the intention of Primary Respiration.

Phase Two is about communication with the natural laws of healing that surround activity at 2 to 3 cycles per minute. We synchronize with the breathing of Primary Respiration and also add the skill of sensing the fulcrum, the Stillness through which the breathing creates form and function. It is a different kind of synchronization from that in Phase One, shifting our awareness more deeply. As this occurs, the treatment automatically expresses itself. The end point of treatment, when compared with Phase One, reveals several differences. We find this kind of synchronization works exclusively with the fluid body and the outcome of treatment is more complete than when working with tissue alone.

Phase Three is centered around the activities of the Long Tide (100 second cycle). We explore an indwelling therapeutic force already present in the lesion field. We learn that the dural system is not made-up of three sickles but rather a series of folds in a sac, arising during growth and development. We see the relationship between the upper and lower dural sacs, awakening us to the independence of two separate tentorium cerebelli. We discover that zone D, the horizon, and the Wire (along which the Long Tide moves during its intended therapeutic course) are all linked as natural laws pertaining to this level of Primary Respiration.

Phase Four focuses on the Midline, a place where the spatial relationships are expressed as a whole. It synchronizes and centers us in such a way that we become aware of Zone D and the Dynamic Stillness. The Third Level Stillness in Phase Four is different from the Stillness in the other Phases – we are centered by the Stillness at the center of creation. Our intention is replaced by the intention of the Tide which can facilitate our spiritual path.

Phase Five is about *the face*. As we approach the face, we use all of the principles that we have learned in Phase One, Two, Three, and Four. We work with automatic shifting and notice differences from how the face is viewed by older models within Osteopathy in the Cranial Field. As we synchronize with the therapeutic presence of the Long Tide we see what we can learn about the face from that landscape. We also work with Seams, Dynamic Stillness, and Ignition.

Phase Six is a continuation of our journey into the Wholeness that generates life and delivers therapeutic forces that transmute lesions once Neutral is expressed. It is a mixture of activities centered around the outside presence of Primary Respiration as something that is a non-biological force and that has a persona. We will also continue to explore seams and then move on to the extremities, first in the embryological terms and then as Sutherland taught them in his work called PowerPoints. Phase 6 is a time to build your understanding of the Tide and refine your skills.

Phase Seven highlights the Health. Dr. Still's famous comment "Find the Health; anyone can find disease," has plagued many minds over the last century. We come to the clear vision of several indwelling aspects of the Health: Love ... liquid light ... and a diamond matrix. A approach to the terminally ill and dying patient is addressed. In the somatic sensation of the Tide passing through the House Under the Sea, our awareness is transmuted by the Health. The lesion is seen as a precognitive act of the Health. Thoracic Respiration, Primary Respiration, and Ignition are as One. The landscape is vast ... and the principles of healing are even more substantial than we have previously experienced..

Phase Eight is a deeper exploration of seams, balanced rhythmic interchange, and the Flame of Intention as a therapeutic modality. Phase Eight is the culmination of our awareness of Wholeness, and ultimately brings us to the Divine Presence, Unconditional Love and Oneness. The living Tide dominates the awareness while forms move to the background. One feels the Breath of Creation in oneself as the Center of Wholeness. One feels the Unfoldment of oneself as one is Created. Our consciousness is a gift; we do not own it and if we try to control it we lose Wholeness.

Phase Nine is when we are able to fully evaluate and treat the Central Nervous System and the Eye. We also address Fire and the therapeutic modality of the Shakedown. True action is moved from Love and makes our perception exist. This Love is self-emptying and by its nature allows us to Serve as part of the Perfect. Perception can be used to Serve something other than ourselves. We have attempted to enter this balance point between the Perfect and the Disease ... it is a point where the whole of everything is suspended by Love as it works to incarnate the Complete. In the balance point of everything is The Intention of the Tide following the movement of the distortion back to a True relationship with the Blueprint of Life.

Pediatrics One explores how children grow as a whole, not in parts as we sometimes believe. Children live in the Direction of Ease of motion present in their fluid metabolic fields, otherwise they get uncomfortable and require assistance. Does your treatment directly support the whole, or does it assume to support the whole? We realize children are not adults and cannot be treated as adults are. We approach the therapeutic modality of the "Meeting Place", prenatal and postnatal periods, the treatment of the pelvis during pregnancy, fetal malposition and labor.

Pediatrics Two is where we deepen in the perceptive awareness necessary to approach the treatment of children. We deepen in our appreciation of Wholeness, the three levels of Stillness and the "Meeting Place". We approach "Desert Neutral", where therapeutics pass into the neutral substance, and a mystery unfolds as the breath of Divine love cascades as a therapeutic force across a night desert landscape, filling and leaving behind no visible effects. We further address treatment of the pelvis and the uterus during pregnancy. We explore thoracic and Primary Respiration in children, and the Family Circle.

Pediatrics Three is where we continue to study the therapeutic Flow of Attention. We deepen in Third Level Stillness and the Meeting Place. The Meeting Place is easily misinterpreted ... our observer must be so still and neutral that the process can be seen as it happens. The central nervous system in the child can be finally approached for evaluation and treatment. We explore teething and also the "locked up head". We use the therapeutic modality of the Flame of Intention, and its connection to the Breath of Life. Everything is transparent to the Breath of Life.

ABOUT THE AUTHOR

James Jealous, D.O. (1943–2021), was an osteopathic physician, teacher, and writer. His life's work was founding and developing **Biodynamics of Osteopathy**, a unique methodology he established within the field of osteopathy, following the lineage of Dr. A.T. Still and Dr. W.G. Sutherland.

He was born in Saco, Maine, and since his father was an osteopathic physician, he was around osteopathy from an early age. He studied at Kirksville College of Osteopathic Medicine in Missouri (now the A.T. Still University of Health Sciences), graduating in 1970. He then set up practice in rural Maine as an osteopathic primary care physician.

Over time, Dr. Jealous saw parallels between the work of embryologist Dr. Erich Blechschmidt and that of osteopathic physician Dr. William Garner Sutherland. This inspiration led him to create his own body of work. In the early 1990s, he began teaching "A Biodynamic View of Osteopathy in the Cranial Field," which, as he developed his specific methodology, was refined to "Biodynamics of Osteopathy."

A deeply spiritual person, he felt most at home in the natural world and was an avid fisherman and hiker.

For more information, please visit:

https://BiodynamicsOfOsteopathy.com

There is a wind passing through ...
it is the motion of creation,
the eternal motion of Divine love.